UNDERSTANDING

BIOTIN

AND BENEFITS

Unlocking Radiant Health: The Comprehensive Guide to Harness the Power of Hair Growth, Glowing Skin, and Nails, Boost Energy, and Support Overall Well-being

DR. LACEY MICHELLE

Disclaimer:

The information provided in this book is for general informational purposes only and is not intended as medical advice.

Readers are encouraged to consult with a qualified healthcare professional for any health concerns or questions.

The author of this book is not affiliated with any individual, website, organization, or products mentioned within.

This book does not endorse or promote any specific brands, services, or external entities. Any references made are purely for illustrative purposes and should not be construed as endorsements.

Readers are responsible for their own decisions and should conduct their own research before making any health-related choices.

Any liability resulting from the use of this information, whether direct or indirect, is disclaimed by the author and publisher.

Contents

Introduction

This book explores the intriguing realm of biotin, an essential nutrient that affects many facets of our health and well-being. It seeks to give readers a thorough grasp of biotin, its significance, sources, and range of applications in areas like metabolism, diabetes control, hair and skin health, and even during pregnancy through its well-organized chapters.

Furthermore, it will help you choose the best biotin supplement for your individual needs, dispel common misconceptions, and offer advice on how to include biotin into your daily routine.

What Is Biotin?

This chapter will examine the principles of biotin, helping you to comprehend its function in the human body, its natural occurrences worldwide, and its historical relevance.

Biotin's Significance

An in-depth discussion of biotin's role in preserving our general health is covered. It discusses the function of biotin in the body, the dangers of a deficit, and the daily amount that is advised for good health.

Biotin Sources

The several sources of biotin, such as foods found naturally, supplements, and goods enhanced with biotin, will be revealed to readers, who will also get a better knowledge of how to include it in their diet.

Hair Health and Biotin

The relationship between biotin and hair health is the main topic of this chapter. It covers how biotin can prevent hair loss, encourage hair growth, and be found in hair care products.

Skin Health and Biotin

Examines topical biotin applications and biotin's effects on skin health, from preserving healthy skin to its potential in controlling acne.

Health of Nails and Biotin

The benefits of biotin for strong, healthy nails are examined, along with how biotin can help prevent brittle nails and if nail care products include biotin.

Metabolism and Biotin

Centers on the metabolism of biotin and discusses its importance for energy production, weight control, and general metabolic processes.

Diabetes and Biotin

The relationship between biotin and diabetes is discussed in this chapter, along with how it affects blood sugar regulation if it can be used as a supplemental medicine and a summary of pertinent studies and research.

Pregnancy and Biotin

Pregnancy-related biotin requirements are discussed, along with possible advantages for the mother and unborn child and safety advice.

Supplemental Biotin

Several forms of biotin supplements, dosage recommendations, and possible adverse effects are covered, giving readers the knowledge they need to make wise choices.

Selecting the Appropriate Biotin Supplement

With an emphasis on important considerations, the value of reading labels, and evaluating the quality and purity of biotin supplements, in navigating the selection process.

Myths and Facts About Biotin

common misconceptions about biotin are dispelled and replaced with assertions backed by science and an awareness of the potential benefits of biotin supplementation.

Your Health and Biotin

This chapter discusses safety measures, how biotin interacts with drugs, and why it's crucial to speak with healthcare professionals before beginning a biotin supplementation regimen.

Including Biotin in Your Daily Routine

Readers will learn doable strategies for incorporating biotin into their daily routines, such as dishes high in nutrients, advice on maintaining healthy skin, hair, and nails, and cultivating a general sense of well-being.

Wrap-Up

The last chapter provides readers with a summary of the advantages of biotin as well as an outlook on upcoming studies and developments related to this crucial supplement.

It is a thorough manual for maximizing biotin's potential for better health and well-being.

CHAPTER ONE

What Is Biotin

Biotin, a water-soluble B-complex vitamin commonly referred to as vitamin H or coenzyme R, is necessary for a number of the body's metabolic functions. It is essential for sustaining healthy skin, hair, and nails as well as for turning food into energy.

A naturally occurring substance, biotin is essential for preserving general health. We shall examine the importance of biotin in the body and its function in several physiological processes in this overview.

Overview:

A member of the B-vitamin family, biotin is essential for a number of the body's biochemical processes. Its main role is as a cofactor for enzymes that are involved in the metabolism of proteins, lipids, and carbohydrates.

For the body to be able to use these macronutrients as energy, this vitamin is necessary.

Furthermore, the production of glucose, amino acids, and fatty acids depends on biotin. It is also essential for preserving the integrity of our nails, hair, and skin.

CHAPTER TWO

Biotin's Significance To The Body:

Energy Metabolism: The synthesis of energy depends heavily on biotin. It aids in the digestion of proteins, lipids, and carbs so that ATP (adenosine triphosphate), the main energy unit of cells, can be produced. Enzymes that are dependent on biotin are engaged in several metabolic processes, including the citric acid cycle, fatty acid synthesis, and glycolysis.

Skin, Hair, and Nails: The promotion of healthy skin, hair, and nails is a common attribute of biotin.

It contributes to the synthesis of keratin, the structural protein that builds these tissues. Sustaining the strength, texture, and general well-being of the skin, hair, and nails requires sufficient quantities of biotin. Supplements containing biotin are occasionally used to treat hair loss and brittle nails.

DNA Synthesis and Repair: The mechanisms of DNA replication and repair also involve biotin. It is essential for preserving the integrity of our cells' genetic material. This role is critical for the body's development and growth, as well as for preventing cellular damage and mutations.

Blood Sugar Regulation: By supporting insulin in its work, biotin helps to keep blood sugar levels under control. The process of transferring glucose from the bloodstream into cells is carried out by insulin. Biotin is crucial for those with diabetes or insulin resistance because it plays a role in the creation of enzymes that facilitate this process.

Neurological Function:

Biotin is thought to be crucial for healthy nerve function, even though its precise involvement in neurological function is not entirely understood. Neurological symptoms like depression, sluggishness, and tingling or numbness in the extremities might result from a biotin deficit.

Pregnancy And Fetal Development:

Pregnant women require increased amounts of the vitamin biotin to promote the growth of the unborn child. This vitamin is vital for fetal development. It is essential for the nervous system and general health development of the infant.

A vital nutrient, biotin is involved in many different metabolic reactions in the body. It's critical for energy metabolism, DNA replication and repair, healthy skin, hair, and nails, blood sugar control, brain function, and fetal development during pregnancy.

Even though biotin shortage is uncommon, maintaining general health and well-being requires making sure you get enough of this vitamin via a balanced diet or supplements.

CHAPTER THREE

Food Sources Of Biotin:

Biotin, sometimes referred to as vitamin B7 or vitamin H, is a water-soluble B vitamin that is essential for several bodily metabolic functions. It is necessary for the body to convert food into energy and to keep skin, hair, and nails healthy. The fact that the body is unable to synthesize biotin means that it needs to be taken from food or supplements, which is one of its most significant characteristics.

Foods Naturally Packed With Biotin:

Many people get their daily recommended dosage of this important vitamin from their diet. Biotin may be found in a wide range of foods.

Egg yolks, liver, nuts, seeds, and some vegetables including spinach and sweet potatoes are some of the main food sources of biotin.

Furthermore, meats, seafood, beans, and some dairy items including milk and cheese contain biotin. Even though the levels of biotin in these foods vary, including them in your diet can help you consume more biotin overall. It is noteworthy that the level of biotin in these meals is not greatly diminished by heating or processing because biotin is heat-stable.

Suggested Daily Intake:

Depending on factors such as age, gender, and stage of life, different amounts of biotin should be consumed each day. However, in general, not much. The recommended daily amount (RDA) for biotin in humans is around 30 micrograms (mcg). The recommended daily dosage for pregnant and nursing women is between 35 and 40 mcg; these quantities may be slightly greater for them.

It's important to remember that most people have relatively low requirements for biotin, and they often get enough from their usual diet. But some things can make you need more biotin than others.

For example, smoking and drinking too much alcohol can lower your body's levels of biotin. Furthermore, a few diseases and drugs may prevent the body from absorbing biotin, which could result in deficits. In some situations, supplementation can be required under a doctor's supervision.

Supplements containing biotin are widely accessible over-the-counter and frequently seen in multivitamin combinations. Even though they are not common, biotin deficits can cause symptoms like skin rashes, hair loss, and neurological problems. For an appropriate diagnosis and supplementation advice, it is best to speak with a healthcare professional if someone has particular health concerns or feels they may be deficient in biotin.

All things considered, the most natural and efficient method of fulfilling your daily needs for biotin is to consume a diversified and balanced diet, which will ensure the correct operation of metabolic processes and the preservation of good skin, hair, and nails.

Insufficient Biotin

Vitamin H, or B7, is another name for biotin, a water-soluble B-complex vitamin that is essential to several bodily metabolic functions. The main function of biotin is in the metabolism of macronutrients, mainly proteins, lipids, and carbs. It facilitates the actions of several significant enzymes by acting as a cofactor. Biotin shortage is a condition caused by a lack of biotin that can negatively impact many body systems.

Symptoms And Indices

A lack of biotin can cause a variety of symptoms and indicators, most of which are related to how the vitamin functions in cellular and energy metabolism. Typical signs of insufficient biotin include:

CHAPTER FOUR

Hair And Skin Issues:

Hair thinning or loss is one of the most obvious signs of a biotin deficiency. It may also result in scaly, dry skin and a rash encircling the lips, nose, and eyes.

Brittle Nails: A lack of biotin can cause nails that are easily broken and brittle.

Three Neurological Problems: People who have a severe biotin deficit may have neurological problems, including sadness, sluggishness, and hallucinations.

Muscle Pain: Since the vitamin is necessary for healthy muscle function, aches, and pains in the muscles may also be an indication of a biotin shortage.

Cardiovascular Issues: Low levels of biotin may exacerbate elevated cholesterol, which may be detrimental to heart health.

Digestive Problems: Inadequate absorption of biotin can result in symptoms of the digestive system, including nausea, vomiting, and diarrhea.

It's important to remember that biotin deficiency is not very prevalent and that many of these symptoms are more frequently linked to other illnesses.

Moreover, the degree of insufficiency can have a significant impact on how severe these symptoms are.

Who's in Danger?

Although biotin deficiency is uncommon, some individuals are more vulnerable than others.

A biotin deficit may be more likely as a result of the following factors:

Genetic Disorders: The body is unable to properly metabolize biotin in certain rare genetic disorders, such as biotinidase deficiency.

To avoid the symptoms of a deficit, people with these diseases need to take supplements of biotin.

Pregnancy and Breastfeeding: Women who are pregnant or nursing may need higher doses of biotin; if they don't get enough of it, they may experience symptoms of deficiency.

Some Medications: Extended use of some medications, like antiepileptic drugs, may cause problems with the absorption and utilization of biotin, which may raise the risk of deficiency.

Overindulgence in Raw Eggs: The protein avidin, found in raw egg whites, can bind to biotin and decrease its absorption. Consuming a large quantity of raw eggs over an extended period might lead to biotin deficiency.

Gastrointestinal illnesses: Individuals with certain gastrointestinal illnesses, such as Crohn's disease or celiac disease, may have decreased biotin absorption, putting them at increased risk.

In most circumstances, a well-balanced diet offers an adequate supply of biotin for the body's needs.

However, persons at risk of biotin shortage, as stated above, may benefit from biotin supplements or dietary modifications to ensure they maintain appropriate biotin levels.

Additionally, it's crucial to consult with a healthcare professional if there are concerns about biotin deficiency or the need for supplementation.

CHAPTER FIVE

Biotin Supplementation

Biotin, also known as vitamin H or B7, is a water-soluble B vitamin that plays a crucial role in various metabolic processes within the body. It is well-known for its essential role in promoting healthy hair, skin, and nails, but it also contributes to the conversion of food into energy and the maintenance of overall well-being.

While biotin is naturally found in many foods, it is also available in supplemental form for those who may have deficiencies or specific health concerns.

Types Of Biotin Supplements

Biotin supplements come in various forms, including capsules, tablets, gummies, and liquid solutions. Each form has its advantages and may be more suitable for different individuals. Capsules and tablets are the most common forms and offer precise dosing.

Biotin gummies, on the other hand, are popular for their palatable taste and can be an attractive option for those who struggle with traditional pill forms.

Liquid biotin supplements are another alternative that allows for easy absorption, but they may require more frequent dosing.

It's important to note that biotin supplements may also be included in multivitamins or other dietary supplements designed to promote overall health and well-being. These combination supplements often contain various vitamins and minerals alongside biotin, offering a comprehensive approach to nutrition.

Recommended Dosages

The recommended daily intake of biotin varies depending on age, sex, and specific dietary needs. Generally, the Recommended Dietary Allowance (RDA) for biotin is 30 micrograms (mcg) per day for adults, with higher requirements during pregnancy and lactation.

However, therapeutic dosages may be higher, particularly for individuals who have biotin deficiency or are using biotin for specific health concerns.

In cases where biotin is taken for its potential benefits on hair, skin, and nails, dosages can range from 5,000 to 10,000 mcg per day, significantly exceeding the RDA.

These higher dosages are often found in biotin supplements marketed to improve the appearance of these features. It is essential to consult with a healthcare professional before exceeding the recommended dosages, as excessive biotin intake may not necessarily yield better results and can pose safety concerns.

Safety And Side Effects

Biotin is generally considered safe when taken within recommended dosages. However, excessive biotin intake can lead to certain side effects.

One common concern is that high doses of biotin can interfere with certain medical tests, such as those used for thyroid function or cardiac markers.

This interference may result in inaccurate test results, so it's crucial to inform healthcare providers if you are taking biotin supplements when undergoing medical testing.

In terms of side effects, biotin is water-soluble, so excess amounts are typically excreted in urine rather than accumulating in the body.

Nonetheless, some individuals may experience side effects, including skin rashes, digestive issues, or changes in insulin sensitivity, particularly when taking very high doses.

It is advisable to monitor for any adverse reactions and seek medical advice if you experience any unusual symptoms while taking biotin supplements.

biotin supplementation offers a convenient way to meet your daily vitamin H needs, especially for those with specific concerns or dietary restrictions.

The choice of biotin supplement form and dosage should be based on individual requirements and preferences, always keeping in mind the importance of following recommended guidelines to ensure safety and effectiveness. If in doubt, consulting with a healthcare professional can provide tailored guidance on the appropriate use of biotin supplements for your unique health and wellness goal.

CHAPTER SIX

Health Benefits Of Biotin

Hair Health: Biotin, also known as vitamin H or B7, is renowned for its role in promoting healthy hair. It is an essential component in the production of keratin, a protein that makes up hair, nails, and the outer layer of the skin. Adequate biotin levels are crucial for maintaining strong and lustrous hair.

Biotin supplements are often recommended to individuals with thinning hair or brittle hair, and they can help improve hair texture and promote hair growth.

Skin Health: Biotin plays a pivotal role in maintaining healthy skin. As part of the B-complex vitamins, it contributes to the synthesis of fatty acids, which are essential for the health of skin cells. Biotin deficiency can lead to skin conditions like dermatitis, dryness, and rashes. The vitamin also supports the body's natural defense mechanisms, helping the skin resist infections and environmental stressors.

Nail Health: Just as it influences hair health, biotin is a key player in maintaining strong and healthy nails. Biotin helps improve nail thickness and prevents brittleness, reducing the likelihood of nail breakage and the development of ridges. Biotin supplements are often recommended to those experiencing weak or peeling nails.

Metabolism and Weight Management: Biotin is essential for various metabolic processes in the body. It helps in the conversion of food into energy by assisting enzymes that break down carbohydrates, fats, and proteins. This metabolic support can have indirect benefits for weight management. While biotin supplements on their own are not a weight loss solution, they can aid in overall metabolic health, potentially contributing to weight control and energy levels.

Diabetes and Blood Sugar Control: Biotin may play a role in blood sugar control and diabetes management. Some research suggests that biotin supplementation can help lower blood glucose levels in people with type 2 diabetes. Biotin may enhance insulin sensitivity and improve glucose utilization, although more studies are needed to establish the full extent of its effectiveness in this regard. Individuals with diabetes need to consult with their healthcare providers before using biotin supplements.

Cognitive Function: While not as well-known for its effects on cognitive function, biotin is a water-soluble B vitamin that participates in various enzymatic reactions. These enzymatic processes are vital for energy production and the overall function of the nervous system. Although biotin deficiency is rare, a shortage of this vitamin may manifest in neurological symptoms, including cognitive impairment. Ensuring adequate biotin intake through a balanced diet or supplementation can contribute to optimal cognitive function.

Biotin is a versatile B vitamin with numerous health benefits. It supports hair, skin, and nail health, aids in metabolism and weight management, may have a role in blood sugar control, and supports cognitive function. While biotin deficiency is uncommon, supplementing with biotin can be beneficial for individuals experiencing issues related to these health aspects. However, it's essential to consult with a healthcare professional before starting any new supplement regimen, especially if you have underlying health conditions or are taking medications that could interact with biotin.

Biotin In Beauty And Cosmetics

Biotin, also known as vitamin H or B7, has gained significant popularity in the world of beauty and cosmetics.

It plays a vital role in promoting healthy skin, hair, and nails, which are essential elements of overall beauty and appearance. Biotin is a water-soluble B vitamin, and it is considered a key component of the B-complex family of vitamins. While its primary function is to assist the body in converting food into energy, it has become a valuable ingredient in various beauty products due to its potential benefits for the external aspects of beauty.

Biotin In Hair Care Products

Hair care products often feature biotin as a prominent ingredient, and for good reason. Biotin is believed to strengthen hair, promote hair growth, and improve hair health.

One of the reasons behind this is that biotin helps in the synthesis of keratin, a protein that makes up the structural foundation of hair. As a result, regular use of biotin-enriched shampoos, conditioners, and hair treatments can contribute to thicker, stronger, and shinier hair.

People with biotin deficiencies may experience hair thinning and brittleness, making biotin supplementation through hair care products particularly beneficial.

Biotin In Skincare Products

Biotin's role in skincare is equally significant. It is known to help maintain healthy skin, primarily through its involvement in fatty acid synthesis.

Healthy fats are essential for maintaining the skin's protective barrier and retaining moisture, which is crucial for preventing dryness and skin issues. Biotin-enriched skincare products, such as creams and serums, aim to support this process by enhancing the skin's overall health and appearance.

They can potentially reduce redness, inflammation, and skin flakiness while promoting a smoother, more radiant complexion.

Nail Care Products With Biotin

Nail health is another aspect of beauty where biotin plays a key role. Biotin is believed to contribute to stronger and more resilient nails. Like with hair, biotin supports the production of keratin in the nails, which helps prevent brittleness and breakage.

Nail care products with biotin may be formulated to provide direct nourishment to the nail bed, promoting healthy and well-manicured nails.

Additionally, individuals with biotin deficiencies may experience nail problems like ridges and thinning, making biotin supplementation an attractive option for improving nail health.

It's important to note that while biotin has gained popularity in beauty and cosmetic products, its effectiveness may vary among individuals, and its impact largely depends on the presence of biotin deficiency. People with healthy diets that include adequate levels of biotin may not experience significant improvements in their hair, skin, or nails by simply using biotin-enriched products. Nonetheless, biotin continues to be a sought-after ingredient in the beauty industry, providing potential benefits to those looking to enhance their external appearance and maintain overall beauty.

Consulting with a healthcare professional or dermatologist is advisable before incorporating biotin-enriched products into your beauty regimen, especially if you suspect a deficiency or have concerns about their efficacy for your specific needs.

CHAPTER SEVEN

Biotin In Medical Treatments

Biotin, also known as vitamin B7 or vitamin H, is a water-soluble B-complex vitamin that plays a crucial role in various biochemical processes in the human body. It is well-known for its involvement in maintaining healthy hair, skin, and nails.

Beyond its cosmetic benefits, biotin has gained attention in the field of medicine for its potential therapeutic applications in treating certain health conditions. Biotin supplements have become increasingly popular, and they are readily available over the counter.

While biotin is essential for overall health, its role in specific medical treatments and its efficacy in addressing various health conditions are subjects of ongoing research and clinical studies.

Biotin For Treating Certain Health Conditions

One of the primary health conditions for which biotin supplementation has gained attention is biotin deficiency. Biotin deficiency is relatively rare, but when it occurs, it can lead to a range of symptoms, including hair loss, brittle nails, skin rashes, and neurological abnormalities.

In severe cases, biotin deficiency can even lead to life-threatening conditions. Supplementing with biotin can effectively address these symptoms and restore normal biotin levels in the body.

Moreover, biotin has been investigated for its potential role in the management of certain metabolic disorders. Biotin-dependent carboxylases, enzymes that require biotin as a cofactor, are essential for various metabolic processes, including fatty acid synthesis and energy production.

Disorders such as biotinidase deficiency and holocarboxylase synthetase deficiency can impair these processes, and supplementation with biotin has been shown to improve the clinical outcomes of affected individuals.

Additionally, biotin has been explored as a potential adjunct therapy for individuals with type 2 diabetes.

Research suggests that biotin may enhance glucose metabolism by stimulating the activity of certain enzymes involved in insulin signaling pathways.

However, the role of biotin in diabetes management is still under investigation, and more research is needed to determine its precise impact on glycemic control.

Research And Clinical Studies

The use of biotin in medical treatments has prompted significant research and clinical studies to better understand its efficacy and safety.

Biotin supplements are generally considered safe when used at recommended doses, but the existing body of research is mixed regarding its effectiveness in addressing certain health conditions.

In the case of biotin deficiency, studies have shown that supplementation can rapidly improve symptoms and restore normal biotin levels in the body.

However, it is essential to diagnose and treat biotin deficiency under the guidance of a healthcare professional to prevent misdiagnosis and unnecessary supplementation.

Research on biotin's role in metabolic disorders has yielded promising results, especially for disorders like biotinidase deficiency.

Clinical trials and case studies have demonstrated significant improvements in affected individuals when biotin supplementation is administered as part of their treatment regimen.

Regarding biotin's potential role in diabetes management, studies have produced mixed outcomes.

Some have suggested a positive impact on glycemic control, while others have not found a significant effect.

This discrepancy underscores the need for further research to elucidate the mechanisms through which biotin may influence glucose metabolism and to identify the specific patient populations that may benefit from biotin supplementation.

while biotin has well-established roles in maintaining healthy hair, skin, and nails, its application in medical treatments is a subject of ongoing research and clinical studies.

Biotin deficiency and certain metabolic disorders have shown promising responses to biotin supplementation, emphasizing its potential therapeutic value.

However, for patients considering biotin supplements for health conditions, it is crucial to consult with a healthcare professional to ensure accurate diagnosis and appropriate treatment. Further research is needed to fully understand the scope of biotin's medical applications and its efficacy in addressing various health conditions.

CHAPTER EIGHT

Biotin And Medication Interactions:

Biotin, also known as vitamin H or B7, is a water-soluble B vitamin that plays a crucial role in various metabolic processes in the human body.

It is commonly found in a variety of foods and is also available as a dietary supplement. While biotin is generally considered safe, there are some important considerations regarding its interactions with medications.

One of the significant interactions between biotin and medications relates to laboratory test results. Biotin can interfere with certain blood tests, particularly those that utilize biotin-dependent enzymes.

These tests include assays for thyroid hormones, troponin (a marker for heart damage), and various hormone and tumor marker tests. When individuals taking biotin supplements undergo these tests, the results may be inaccurate or misleading. This interference can potentially lead to misdiagnosis and inappropriate medical decisions.

To avoid such interactions, healthcare providers must be informed about biotin supplement use in their patients.

Patients should also disclose their biotin intake to their healthcare providers before undergoing any blood tests to ensure accurate results.

In some cases, patients may be advised to discontinue biotin supplementation for a specific period before undergoing such tests.

How It Affect The Blood Sugar Regulation

Another medication interaction to consider is related to anticonvulsant drugs, primarily phenobarbital and phenytoin. These medications can reduce biotin levels in the body.

Therefore, individuals taking anticonvulsants, especially for extended periods, may be at risk of biotin deficiency.

Healthcare providers should monitor biotin status in such patients and recommend biotin supplementation if necessary to prevent deficiency.

It's essential to note that biotin is generally well-tolerated when taken at recommended doses, and most people do not experience adverse interactions with common medications.

However, it's always wise to consult with a healthcare provider when considering biotin supplementation, especially if you are taking prescription medications to ensure there are no potential interactions that could affect your health or the accuracy of medical tests.

Special Considerations For Certain Groups:

While biotin is considered safe for the majority of the population when taken at recommended doses, there are specific groups for whom special considerations should be made regarding biotin supplementation.

Pregnant and breastfeeding women, for instance, have increased biotin requirements. Biotin is essential for fetal development and the health of the mother during pregnancy and lactation.

However, it's generally recommended to obtain these increased biotin needs through a balanced diet rather than high-dose supplements.

If biotin supplementation is deemed necessary for pregnant or breastfeeding women, it should be done under the guidance of a healthcare provider to ensure safety and efficacy.

Individuals with certain medical conditions, such as diabetes, multiple sclerosis, or hereditary disorders affecting biotin metabolism, may require special attention when it comes to biotin supplementation.

In some cases, biotin supplementation may be recommended as part of their medical management, while in others, it could potentially interfere with existing treatments.

Healthcare providers should be aware of these considerations and make appropriate recommendations based on the individual's medical history and needs.

Additionally, individuals with a history of allergies or hypersensitivity to biotin should exercise caution when considering biotin supplementation.

Allergic reactions to biotin supplements are rare but can be severe. Individuals in this category should consult with a healthcare provider before starting any biotin supplementation.

Biotin is an essential B vitamin that plays a significant role in various bodily functions. While it is generally safe for the general population, individuals should be aware of its potential interactions with medications and specific considerations for certain groups, as outlined above.

It is always recommended to consult with a healthcare provider before initiating biotin supplementation to ensure its safety and appropriateness for one's circumstances.

CHAPTER NINE

Biotin In Pregnancy And Breastfeeding

Biotin, also known as vitamin H or B7, is a water-soluble B vitamin essential for various metabolic processes in the human body.

It plays a crucial role in maintaining healthy skin, hair, and nails, as well as assisting in the metabolism of fats, carbohydrates, and amino acids.

While biotin is important for general health, its significance is particularly pronounced during pregnancy and breastfeeding, as it is involved in critical processes related to fetal development and maternal well-being.

Biotin Requirements During Pregnancy

Pregnancy is a time when the demand for many nutrients, including biotin, increases significantly. Biotin is important for the growth and development of the fetus, as it contributes to the formation of the baby's organs and tissues.

During pregnancy, there is a higher demand for biotin because of increased cell division, DNA synthesis, and energy metabolism which are essential for fetal development. Additionally, maternal biotin levels are required to ensure the healthy development of the baby's nervous system.

The recommended daily intake of biotin for pregnant women is typically higher than for non-pregnant individuals.

The exact requirements can vary depending on factors such as age, pre-existing health conditions, and dietary habits. While there isn't a specific daily intake established solely for biotin during pregnancy, it is generally advised that pregnant women should aim for a balanced diet that includes an adequate amount of biotin-rich foods. This can be achieved by consuming foods like eggs, nuts, seeds, and dairy products, which are natural sources of biotin.

In some cases, healthcare providers may recommend biotin supplementation during pregnancy, especially if a pregnant woman has specific health issues or dietary restrictions that might hinder the intake of biotin through food alone. However, pregnant women must consult their healthcare professionals before taking any supplements to determine the appropriate dosage and to ensure that they don't exceed safe levels.

Safety Of Biotin Supplementation

Biotin supplementation is generally considered safe for most individuals when taken within recommended daily limits. However, as with any dietary supplement, it is important to exercise caution during pregnancy. While biotin is a water-soluble vitamin and excess amounts are typically excreted in urine, there are potential risks associated with excessive biotin intake.

One concern with excessive biotin supplementation during pregnancy is the potential to interfere with certain laboratory tests, such as those used to diagnose conditions like hypothyroidism and gestational diabetes. Biotin supplements can lead to false positive or false negative results in these tests, which could have significant implications for maternal and fetal health.

Pregnant women need to discuss biotin supplementation with their healthcare provider to ensure it is both necessary and safe.

They can guide women on appropriate dosages and timing, taking into account the individual's specific health status.

 A well-balanced diet that includes a variety of nutrient-rich foods remains the primary means to meet biotin requirements during pregnancy, with supplementation being considered only when necessary.

biotin is a vital nutrient during pregnancy and breastfeeding due to its role in fetal development and maternal health.

The requirements for biotin increase during pregnancy, and it is important for pregnant women to ensure they meet their dietary needs.

Biotin supplementation may be recommended in certain cases, but it should be approached with caution and only under the guidance of a healthcare provider to ensure safety and effectiveness while avoiding potential interference with diagnostic tests. Prioritizing a healthy and balanced diet remains the cornerstone of ensuring adequate biotin intake during these critical life stages.

CHAPTER TEN

Biotin Myths And Facts: Debunking Common Misconceptions - Separating Fact From Fiction

Biotin, also known as vitamin H or B7, is a water-soluble B vitamin that plays a crucial role in various bodily functions. It is often touted as a remedy for hair, skin, and nail health and is a popular dietary supplement. However, there are numerous myths and misconceptions surrounding biotin, which can lead to confusion and misunderstanding about its actual benefits and limitations. In this discussion, we aim to clarify the myths and facts surrounding biotin, separating fiction from scientific reality.

Common Misconception

One common myth about biotin is that it is a miracle solution for hair loss and hair growth.

While biotin is essential for the maintenance of healthy hair, skin, and nails, it does not possess magical properties that can instantly reverse hair loss or significantly accelerate hair growth. Hair loss can result from various factors, including genetics, hormonal imbalances, and medical conditions, and biotin alone is unlikely to address these underlying issues.

Biotin supplements may help individuals with biotin deficiencies, but they should not be considered a universal remedy for hair-related concerns.

Another widespread misconception is that biotin can prevent or cure acne. Some people believe that taking biotin supplements can improve their skin health and reduce acne breakouts. However, scientific evidence to support this claim is limited. While biotin is essential for overall skin health, excessive biotin intake can sometimes lead to skin issues. Therefore, it's essential to maintain a balanced intake and consult with a healthcare professional before using biotin for skin-related concerns.

Awareness And Potential Benefits

Furthermore, there is a myth that taking high doses of biotin is safe and beneficial. In reality, biotin is a water-soluble vitamin, meaning excess amounts are typically excreted in the urine. However, taking extremely high doses of biotin supplements, often exceeding recommended daily values, can lead to potential side effects and interfere with certain medical tests. Biotin can interfere with lab results, including thyroid function tests and cardiac biomarker tests, potentially leading to inaccurate diagnoses. Therefore, it's crucial to use biotin supplements as directed and avoid excessive intake.

On the other hand, it is a fact that biotin is vital for various biochemical processes in the body. It plays a key role in metabolizing macronutrients, particularly carbohydrates, proteins, and fats, which are essential for energy production and overall health. Biotin is also essential for the synthesis of fatty acids and the formation of glucose, contributing to the proper functioning of the nervous system. This makes it a critical nutrient for maintaining general well-being.

Another fact is that biotin deficiency is relatively rare. Most people obtain an adequate amount of biotin through their regular diet, as it is found in a variety of foods such as eggs, nuts, seeds, and certain vegetables. Biotin deficiency is primarily associated with specific medical conditions or genetic disorders that impair biotin absorption. In such cases, biotin supplementation is recommended under the guidance of a healthcare professional.

it is essential to distinguish between the myths and facts surrounding biotin. While biotin is undoubtedly essential for the maintenance of healthy hair, skin, and nails, it is not a panacea for all related concerns. Biotin supplements should be used judiciously and as directed, and individuals should consult with healthcare professionals for personalized advice. Understanding the limitations and benefits of biotin can help individuals make informed decisions about its use and avoid falling prey to common misconceptions.

CHAPTER ELEVEN

Choosing The Right Biotin Supplement

Biotin, also known as vitamin B7 or vitamin H, is a water-soluble B vitamin that plays a crucial role in various metabolic processes within the human body.

It is essential for the metabolism of carbohydrates, fats, and proteins, and it also contributes to the health of our hair, skin, and nails. Biotin is naturally present in many meals, and our bodies can also create it in the gut through the activities of specific bacteria. However, in some situations, individuals may require biotin supplements to maintain their health or correct specific inadequacies.

Factors To Consider

When considering the use of biotin supplements, it's crucial to make informed selections to ensure that you are getting the best product for your needs. Here are some crucial variables to consider:

Biotin Dosage: The first and most important consideration is the dosage. Biotin supplements are available in various quantities, often ranging from 1,000 to 10,000 micrograms (mcg) per serving. The optimum dosage depends on your specific needs and the reason for taking the supplement. For example, those with a documented biotin deficiency may require a greater dosage, while individuals aiming to improve hair and nail health might opt for lower levels.

Form of Biotin: Biotin supplements are available in numerous forms, such as biotin capsules, soft gels, gummies, and even biotin-infused shampoos or lotions. The choice of form relies on personal preference and ease of intake. Some people may find candies or liquid versions more appetizing, while others prefer classic capsules or soft gels.

Purity and Quality: Ensuring the purity and quality of the biotin supplement is vital. Look for products that are created by reputed brands and meet high-quality control requirements. Independent third-party testing can provide an extra level of assurance regarding the supplement's potency and purity.

Bioavailability: D- and DL-biotin are two of the types of biotin supplements that are available. The naturally occurring version, D-biotin, is thought to be more efficient and bioavailable. Selecting D-biotin-containing supplements may increase its efficacy.

Extra constituents: Other vitamins, minerals, or herbal extracts are possible extra constituents in certain biotin pills. These may offer supplementary advantages, but it's crucial to be sure they complement any other supplements you may be taking and your health objectives. Furthermore, exercise caution around any substances or allergens you might wish to stay away from.

Allergies and Dietary Limitations: It's critical to thoroughly review the components of any supplement you are taking if you have any food allergies or dietary limitations. Supplements containing biotin could include chemicals or fillers that are problematic for people with certain dietary restrictions or allergies.

CHAPTER TWELVE

Examining Supplement Labelling

Selecting the appropriate biotin supplement requires carefully reading the label. The following are some things to consider:

Serving Size:

To calculate the dosage, check the suggested serving size and the amount of biotin per serving.

Purity: Verify the product's absence of pollutants and impurities by looking for any quality certificates or independent testing results.

• Form of Biotin: Find out which particular form of biotin is included in the supplement; D-biotin is usually preferred.

• Expiration Date: To guarantee the potency and efficacy of the supplement, always check its expiration date.

• Use guidelines: Adhere to the suggested dosage and usage directions listed on the package.

• Other Ingredients: If the supplement includes other ingredients, carefully consider how well they match your nutritional goals and preferences.

In conclusion, careful examination of elements including dosage, form, purity, quality, and the presence of other substances is necessary when choosing the best biotin supplement. To make an informed choice and make sure the selected product satisfies your unique needs and preferences, you must read the labels on supplements. To find the right amount of biotin to take on an individual basis, it is best to speak with a healthcare provider or nutritionist. They can offer tailored advice based on your unique health and wellness objectives.

CHAPTER THIRTEEN

Including Biotin In Your Daily Routine For Health

Including biotin, sometimes referred to as vitamin B7 or vitamin H, in your daily routine can have several positive effects on your general health. Water-soluble vitamin B-tin is essential for several body processes, including the metabolism of proteins, lipids, and carbohydrates.

This vitamin is involved in the synthesis of fatty acids, amino acids, and glucose and is necessary for keeping healthy skin, hair, and nails. Including biotin in your daily routine can be beneficial whether your goals are to maintain your metabolic processes or to enhance the health of your skin, hair, and nails.

When adding biotin to your daily routine for health, there are a few critical things to keep in mind to get the best effects. Before beginning any new supplementation, it is first and foremost recommended that you speak with a medical practitioner or a qualified dietician.

They can offer advice on the proper dosage and any interactions with other vitamins or drugs you may be taking.

You can select the type of biotin supplement that best fits your needs and preferences from a variety of formats, including gummies, tablets, and capsules.

Since biotin is a water-soluble vitamin that the body cannot retain for long, taking it consistently is essential. This indicates that to maintain adequate levels, a daily intake is advised. It's usually not a problem if you skip a dose once in a while, but sticking to a schedule can help you get the most out of your biotin supplements.

The recommended daily allowance (RDA) for biotin is dependent upon several aspects, including age, sex, and life stage, when it comes to dosage. Nonetheless, people should normally strive for a daily intake of around 30 micrograms (mcg).

Those who are nursing or pregnant might need a little bit more. However, it is important to remember not to go beyond the upper consumption amount, which is generally regarded as safe for adults at 5,000 mcg per day, as this could have unfavorable effects.

Combining A Balanced Diet With Biotin

While supplementing with biotin can offer an extra dose of this vital vitamin, it's crucial to keep in mind that a well-balanced diet is the foundation of good health.

Since biotin occurs naturally in a variety of foods, including these in your diet can help guarantee that you get enough of this nutrient.

Eggs, nuts, seeds, whole grains, dairy products, meat, and fish are among the foods high in biotin. Specifically, the yolk of eggs contains a substantial quantity of biotin, making them a good source of this vitamin.

Furthermore, the amount of biotin you consume might be influenced by the bacteria in your stomach that produce biotin.

Choosing a diet that is varied and well-rounded will not only give you biotin but also other vital vitamins and minerals that will benefit your general well-being.

When including biotin into your health regimen, this all-encompassing approach to diet will help you attain greater outcomes.

Additionally, as these parts of your appearance are frequently influenced by your general food choices and lifestyle, they can help support ideal skin, hair, and nail health.

Including biotin in your daily regimen can help you support vital metabolic processes and keep your skin, hair, and nails in good condition.

You may optimize the benefits of this crucial vitamin and enhance your general health by adhering to the guidelines for best outcomes and combining biotin supplementation with a well-balanced diet full of foods high in biotin. Always seek the advice of a healthcare provider for individualized recommendations on diet and supplements to suit your unique requirements and objectives.

CHAPTER FOURTEEN

Biotin And Your General Health

Water-soluble vitamin B-complex biotin, often known as vitamin H or B7, is essential for sustaining general health and well-being.

This vital vitamin is well-known for its participation in several biochemical bodily functions, most notably those connected to metabolism and food-derived energy consumption.

Beyond its involvement in fundamental biological processes, biotin has drawn interest for its possible advantages in advancing a holistic approach to health.

The Comprehensive Method Of Healing

A holistic approach to health emphasizes the connections between different facets of well-being, stressing the interdependence of one's mental, emotional, and physical well-being. It encourages people to strive for complete well-being by taking into account not just their physical health but also their mental and emotional emotions.

Given its ability to address multiple aspects of health at once, biotin falls into this holistic framework.

The Function Of Biotin In General Health
Hair, Skin, and Nails: It's well-known that biotin helps to maintain healthy skin, hair, and nails. It aids in the synthesis of keratin, a protein that gives these tissues their structural integrity.

Sufficient levels of biotin are linked to more resilient hair, less fragile nails, and radiant skin.

Energy Metabolism: Proteins, lipids, and carbs may all be converted into energy more easily when biotin is present. Maintaining adequate energy levels is critical for this function, which in turn supports general vigor and well-being.

Blood Sugar Control: Biotin might also help with blood sugar control.

According to certain research, it enhances insulin sensitivity, which is essential for preserving steady blood glucose levels. Since blood sugar swings can affect mood and energy levels, stable blood sugar is crucial for both physical and mental health.

Brain Health: Biotin is known to be involved in the manufacture of fatty acids, which are necessary for preserving good brain function, while research on its significance in brain health is still in its early stages. Supplementing with biotin may benefit cognitive health, according to preliminary data.

Digestive Health: By aiding in the synthesis of enzymes that aid in the breakdown of food for nutrient absorption, biotin promotes digestive health. Because a healthy digestive system makes sure the body gets the nutrients it needs to function at its best, it is essential to general well-being.

Holistic Beauty: The effects of biotin on nails, skin, and hair go beyond appearance to include emotional stability and self-worth. Mental and emotional well-being can be greatly impacted by one's sense of self-worth.

Conclusion

As an essential B-complex vitamin, biotin has a variety of functions that support general health. Biotin has a significant effect on many different facets of physical health, from improving the condition of hair, skin, and nails to controlling blood sugar and energy metabolism.

Furthermore, its potential benefits for emotional and mental health are becoming more widely acknowledged. Biotin complements the holistic approach to health, which recognizes the interdependence of mental, emotional, and physical states, by treating these various aspects of health. But it's crucial to take a responsible approach to biotin supplementation or dietary inclusion, making sure that it enhances a general healthy lifestyle and dietary decisions.

In the end, biotin is but one crucial component in the larger picture of attaining and preserving complete well-being.